The Secret to Lose Weight

Stop Your Cravings and Flatten Your Belly in a Snap

The Sugar-Candida-yeast link

and the know how to beat obesity.

The Secret to Lose Weight, Stop Your Cravings

and Flatten Your Belly in a Snap

The Secret to Lose Weight

Stop Your Cravings and Flatten Your Belly in a Snap

The Sugar-Candida-yeast link
and the know how to beat obesity.

Ferny Roby

The Secret to Lose Weight, Stop Your Cravings

and Flatten Your Belly in a Snap

Copyright ©2012 F Robaina
ISBN-13:
978-1475269888

ISBN-10:
1475269889

Table of Contents

DON'T GET FAT NO MORE

Find out and program yourself to stop being an eating machine and get in shape right away.

Lets be real, you are fat because you are hungry permanently, it's not a flaw in you, it's not mental, is true Hunger that cries within you. If you are overweight, it's not because you eat too much. it's because you are starving your body on a cellular level. When you don't eat you feel miserable and weak. If you were out of this and get free of this chains and bondage you'll fell like a million dollars and free like a bird. let me explain you why and how:

But before let me tell you this: **If you don't want to read a lot and want to go straight to a guide to do it, or want to live this reading for later go to the last section of this book named "Simple guide to free yourself from Hunger and Cravings and binges." in page 72**

Preface

The basic reason people get overweight is because they are in permanent hunger and cravings. Hunger is defined as a feeling experienced when the glycogen (glucose or sugars) level of the liver falls below a threshold, usually followed by a desire to eat. In other words this means that we feel hungry when our sugars in liver are low. How is it that people who just take a lot of sweet food becomes hungry quickly?

So the question here is why in America, land of food and abundance, there is such a great proportion of craving people?

The Program Basic features

o This Program is different to any other you know. You'll learn the secret in food we eat that makes you overeat. What is the real way to change your body cravings?

o Why is that you are addicted to sugars or any sweet meal.
o The real culprit of American obesity is here described. You will be amazed!
o The reason of overweight is because we become steadily hungry, so we eat and eat again and again and we become a permanent weight gaining eating super machine. Once you know what is causing this condition is very easy to stop it.
o This Program Is based in making you know who the real culprits of constant cravings are.
o This program won't drive you to the crisis where most of the dietsts do, where the bad feeling momentum of low energy makes you quit. What is the real way to change your body cravings?
o
  You will learn several supplements you have not heard of to complement your effort. This supplements can help you cut immediately your sweet craving and binges in a natural effortless and harmless way.
o You learn why is that you are overweight and how to break that condition in *a simple and easy way...*"

o You will eat whatever you want of delicious food and recipes. You'll learn the real principle to get rid of hunger and cravings, and what to pick to eat to maintain your plan.
o You will keep body energy at all times
o You will eat deliciously natural foods and you'll enjoy them at the fullest, even more than the foods, snacks and desserts you crave now and binge for.

o You will learn what to choose in any place, restaurant or fast food zone, to eat, according to this Program.
o This program is designed to activate your liver and thyroid function to its best.

Introduction

The Secret to Lose Weight, Stop Your Cravings
and Flatten Your Belly in a Snap

This work contains a nutritional breakthrough. I am sure you have read a lot about sugar and its side effects and about Candida and other parasites, but the mechanism how you are hungry never has been explained in the way you are going to read here. This knowledge will show you the real and original cause and mechanisms of your hunger and cravings and what is the way to stop it. It will show you the real cause of overweight and fat. When you learn the way things happen is very easy to isolate the culprit and stop it. So please learn how to stop being an Eating Machine!

This information really works. All the people who have applied it had lost many inches out of their waist and shed many pounds off their weight. Once you are on the right path eating correctly you can stay long time doing so without quitting. This ease of use is because this Program works in the critical stages were most of other Programs fail. And secondly because is not a starving diet; you can eat abundantly with guidelines. By following it you will find the power to defeat bloating and inflammation; and a safe and reliable way to lose weight and stay on course.

You can (and must) eat abundantly . There is no hunger involved in this Program. But you will learn what are the nutrients and the know how to help you stop your cravings.

most of the dietsts fail helping you consume your fatty areas. This is because fatty areas are bags of encapsulated toxins. When toxins start breaking make you feel miserably sick and put your liver in jeopardy. This makes you feel weak and sick. At this point most dieters quit. This Program helps you to gain enough thermogenesis trough certain foods and to detoxify and empower your liver. The liver will kick out your fat toxins and your bulk. Your metabolism will gain the ability to produce more heat If you stick to this Program, the breaking point is almost null or non-existent.

Hunger and Cravings

The actual fundamental cause individuals get obese is due to the fact they tend to be in long term craving for food and urges. Hunger is actually identified as a sensation experienced whenever the glycogen (blood sugar level of the liver organ comes under a limit, typically followed by a wish to eat. In other words this indicates that we all feel starving whenever our glucose in liver are reduced. How is it that folks who just get a lot of sweet meals will become famished so rapidly?

So the question the following is exactly why in America, land of food and abundance, presently there is such a fantastic proportion of yearning people? Why glycogen ranges fall swiftly and abruptly in the majority of people? Why many individuals become consuming and fat-gaining machines? The cause is simply one: these people are progressively and completely hungry!

If you feel hungry at all times, you are right and your body is correct! You eat too much because you are hungry, really very hungry. Your corpulence is a reflection of your hunger. There is a deep-rooted cause that triggers these urges. Hunger comes from the deepest in you and without killing the causing agent, hunger will stay for life with you because it has become an ecological and self maintained system in your gut.
You feel hungry because your liver glucose levels become very low and you are feeling real and genuine hunger.

Where lays the cause of your permanent hunger and binges. Getting rid of hunger's real cause. Cause that lays in your guts, your size will reduce as you stop craving food!

What is the real cause of being overweight? How can you get to be able to control the real culprits of your permanent hunger: Parasites? These parasites consume your energy and your willpower. They bring you to hypoglycemia (very low sugar in liver and body) and to adrenal and liver exhaustion. These parasites have made of you a hungry starving bag full of food and counting.

With this nutritional approach you will (and must) eat a lot. You will rip apart your fat without pain. You will destroy the source of your hunger eating correctly. You will succeed.

How is this possible? The answer rests in the following pages.

My story

I was grown with very bad eating habits. My mother had the idea that a kid had to eat all day to be healthy. Each meal was abundant and desserts and cakes were the norm. I had the tendency to eat all day. Since my young adulthood I was heavy like my mother, brothers and sisters and always tried to be slim. I dieted many times and many times failed. Diets take me to the starvation point where I start feeling sick or weak. Suddenly by taking a bit of carbs or a cake bite I felt better and different and all my battles were lost in a second.

These crisis stages were really very critical and made me many times do a yo-yo diet. I need a lot of willpower to start and keep a diet for some time. I had that initial firmness but as soon as I started feeling bad and increasingly weak, pain made me quit. It was a kind of demolishing will torture chamber. At that time my liver was overcrowded after eliminating so many long-time fat encapsulated toxins in my body. Pain and hunger cut out my resolution. I feel weak and sick: hunger and cravings, comfort and release, sugars and cakes were always present, available everywhere...

Most diets take you to a point where you start feeling kind of sick or sluggish and brain fogged and your humour is critical. You start taking foods that rapidly release glucose. These meals are cookies, pasta pizzas doughnuts sugary chocolates or else that make you feel so good that you start loosing all whatever you gained or gaining whatever weight you had lost.

Secondly and most important, I questioned myself if there was something in my mind or body that was making me hungry? Why do I was always obsessed with food? I had always a big appetite and was always craving something. Why was I always desiring of a snack or a sweet something? Why I was eating all day long? It was something wrong in my mind or it was that this urge was coming from somewhere else? The answer that I find to that question made me find an answer to this issue about the way American people eat and a great part of world's population. I found that there was nothing wrong in my mind or psychology or in the mind or millions others who have the same problem and have cravings all the time. There was some inner workings or something real going in my guts demanding me to eat more and more…

There was something –I supposed- that most Americans ate through their regular diet that created a craving monster within . That question was not answered by counting calories or eating less fats or sugars or calories. It was a kind of food enslavement that took me and many other people to an eating to death or suicide scenario. Live to eat not eat to live.

Of course eating lot of fats or Carbs will make anybody overweight. Sure is, that if you eat plenty of calories you will get fat. But being fat is not a mathematical question, the real question is: why are there so many people in America becoming eating machines? In nature, animals will eat plenty when available but never will overeat to be overweight. **Why is that people become addicted to food? The second question is why they become addicted to incorrect food.** That meant that we were eating something incorrect or processing the food in a wrong way that make us get heavy and fat. This is the most important revelation in this book.

Learning who the culprit is in this process, will take you to get rid of this urge to eat that comes directly from your guts and takes control of your brain and will power by the means of pain and hunger.

Learning what is the real cause in this slaving process and how these mechanisms operate makes easy to anybody to handle hunger cravings and control overweight.

When I learned the real cause of my binges and cravings. Immediately I started handling my overweight, and food desires in an easy manner.

All that I found made me certain what is the way to get **slim without pain. Later** I realized that I found in my research **the mechanism of the basic underlying reason for obesity in America,** That many people needed this simple and real solution to escape of food addiction.

When you understand the mechanism of this complicated quiz you'll say: it was so easy!

This approach is different from all others you have read because is showing you the real and essential cause of you being overweight. When you learn the real cause you can take action following the principles underlined here and then get on shape easy and quickly.

You may ask yourself now: what the essential cause of people gaining weight and enslaving to food consumption could be. Is there a real main cause of being overweight? Stopping this causing agent may cut immediately my hunger cravings and binges?

What is the main reason for you, me or anybody to become an eating machine

The main reason of being permanently hungry are parasites. Parasites that we grow in our digestive system. Parasites that we farm and nurture by the way we eat. These parasites become our masters dictating us what to eat and crave to keep feeding them and helping them grow their colonies in our body. These parasites nurtured by the way we were trained to eat by our parents (which had the same story) deep-rooted in our body and body organs will force us to eat an excess of sugars and carbohydrates to first-feed them. After we eat they will consume all the food available in our guts and trigger our hunger and then our craving for more . Secondly they will make us eat whatever is good for them (not for us). This means you will eat to feed them: you will work to feed them: you will rush to the supermarket to buy whatever is good for them. In other words they will be your masters.

In simple words We are eating to keep them fed. We eat that way because we have been slaved by them to feed them. If you think this is an insane affirmation please read the annexed section about parasites.

Parasites taking control of our minds?

Parasites taking control of our mind is nothing strange in the animal world. Look at this parasite story in Discover Magazine, August, 2000:

"The mature lancet fluke, Dicrocoelium dendriticum, nestles in cows and other grazers, which spread the fluke's eggs in their manure. Hungry snails swallow the eggs, which hatch in their intestines. The immature parasites drill through the wall of a snail's gut and settle in the digestive gland. There the flukes produce offspring, which make their way to the surface of the snail's body. The snail tries to defend itself by walling the parasites off in balls of slime, which it then coughs up and leaves behind in the grass."

"Along comes an ant, which swallows a slime ball loaded with hundreds of lancet flukes. The parasites slide down into the ant's gut and then

wonder for a while through its body, eventually moving to the cluster of nerves that control the ant's mandibles. Most of the lancet flukes head back to the abdomen, where they form cysts, but one or two stay behind in the ant's head."

"There the flukes do some parasitic voodoo on their hosts. As the evening approaches and the air cools, the ants find themselves drawn away from their fellows on the ground and upward to the top of a blade of grass. Clamped to the tip of the blade, the infected ant waits to be devoured by a cow or some other grazer passing by."

"If the ant sits the whole night without being eaten and the sun rises, the flukes let the ant loosen its grip on the grass. The ant scurries back down to the ground and spends the day acting like a regular insect again. If the host were to bake in the heat of the direct sun, the parasites would die with it. When evening comes again, they send the ant back up a blade of grass for another try. After the ant finally tumbles into a cow's stomach, the flukes burst out and make their way to the cow's liver, where they will live out their lives as adults."

"The greed for Pane (Bread), Potatoes, Pizza, Pasta the four P Sweets is one of the characteristic symptoms of the Candida infection.

*This particular greed for simple sugars is mediated and motivated by the **79 toxins that monilia (Candida) introduces in the haematic circle**, and which act on the central nervous system modifying the subject thoughts. It is comprehensible why Candida infection is responsible for the chronic fatigue syndrome for the hyperactivity, the depression, the anxiety,the bulimia,and for the anorexia."*[1]

---

[1] *Dr ENZONZO DI MAIO* http://www.psoriasi.org/

When one is in front of a doughnut a soda or an ice cream and can not stop from taking it. How would you call this abduction of your will? Actually something within your body is governing your will, I would say that is a truly parasites governance over one self.

These parasites consume (eat) all our glucose and, as we said before, hunger is a decrease to a certain threshold of available glucose to the body . No matter how much you eat, these parasites will grow more colonies and finish all the food (glucose) you meant was for your body and to get you out of hunger.

hypoglycemia (low glucose or starving situation) will occur each time this parasites eat most of our glucose. Their toxic debris (more than 70 toxins) will inactivate and fatten your liver, pancreas and other organs helping in this weight gaining process.

We are what we eat, The way to eradicate this parasites that we have been talking about: Not feed them with the food they use to grow reproduce and thrive. **Learning how to naturally eradicate these parasites by the way we eat and with help of some natural supplements is the goal of this Program.** This Program is thought in a way to take action starving the ones who starve us. This is through a diet that overrides these parasites and kills them with a vengeance: death by hunger!

II Part

The Cause of Obesity in America (and elsewhere)

Read carefully:

<u>Yeast and Candida ingested and nurtured daily in all type of breads, cakes, doughnuts and cookies plus all food filled with lot of sugars (mostly sodas and liquid beverages) are the main belly boosters in the American diet. And the main cause of obesity in America and elsewhere.</u>

Sugar is the food additive that makes this parasites thrive and govern yourself. 99% of processed foods in the market have extra sugar.

What do this means?
In a shell this is the way you and me and many people have become overweight:

How bread works with our parasites.

Bread is present in 90 % of our daily meals. Bread is made with Yeast which is a parasite ; which expands the dough to a 150 to 300 % in size. In bread production, yeast cells convert carbohydrates into carbon dioxide, which causes the dough to expand or rise As more strong and alive Yeast is in our body the stomach expansion is stronger. They are living and reproductive beings and with sugar they can stay alive and reproduce indefinitely even more if you add more each day as you intake all kinds of bread and pastries with lot of sugars added.

If you put some warm water , yeast and sugar in a jar and you cap it with a balloon , you'll see the balloon inflates totally in about 30 minutes. The same thing happens to your cells and your belly that means strong inflammation.

You want to know what this yeast does in you?

1. Bloating: It boosts your stomach like a balloon and expands it in size. It makes a lot of gas (CO2 carbon dioxide) and alcohol, bloating in the intestine. Worst than that, bloating makes your stomach and your intestine full of gas and food sensors within make you

feel hungry because they only detect air (GAS) surrounding your gastrointestinal body. Additionally you become addicted to the alcohol produced in this interchange.

This means you feel starving being full of food. Your brain sensors feel that there is not food to eat in the stomach walls.

2. Belly expansion makes the stomach bigger and bigger by expanding it at maximum.
    a. Due to stretching of the belly your appetite increasingly looks for more food to feel full.
3. Inflammation: If you eat bread in a Daily basis you are making en expandable balloon of your entire digestive tracts Stomach intestine, etc. This means a constant expanded abnormality. And you'll feel starving! This constant expansion press and damage also inner organs like kidneys heart and liver. This process also increases inflammation that is a pathological stage. Parasite toxin debris produce also inflammation which is the 1st stage for the worst diseases. That means cancers, diabetes and heart thrombosis between others.

4. All these yeast eats all the available glucose in your body. This makes you weak and hungry, because lowers your liver glucose.
5. Will reproduce this bloating mechanism in your cells.

Daily bread eating constructs a yeast ecosystem in your guts that becomes a perfect fat machine. Lets see why:

Yeast Ecosystem

Glucose and Sugars

Glucose is one of the most basic energy factor for living creatures. Cells use it as the source of energy and a metabolic intermediate. Most food converts to glucose and glucose is the medium to have energy to move to think to digest to exercise or to do anything

Glucose is the base for forming the main energy molecule for living beings at the cellular level: ATP. Glucose is obtained from any nutrient it can be simple carbohydrates or a piece of meat. Glucose derived from sucrose (sugar) or breads is a quick available glucose but has many predators in our digestive system.

Glucose must be in your blood so cells can take it and produce energy and allow many biological processes. If glucose doesn't get inside cells you don't get the benefit of it. Glucose is a kind of natural addictive drug for living organisms. Trees use sweet fruits as bait to make other animals move their seeds and expand geographically. Flowers use pollen (sweet) as bait to bees. That is so because glucose has a basic key to neuron and brain pleasure terminals and is the key for the energy to cell's life. Chocolate molecules or cocaine or sugars have a similar kind of that same key in neurons. These are called the opiate terminals in our neural system.

Cells demand of glucose is first priority and that extends to the whole organism itself. We could say that all relations between living creatures are a battle for obtaining glucose from the others. The reason is that glucose is the key ingredient to energy, activity and life itself.

Our energy depends of glucose. All types of food must be converted in glucose so energy may be reached by cells.

Digestion of Proteins and vegetables produce long lasting glucose in blood and this glucose is hidden through glycols and is not edible for yeast and Candida. So all the energy they contain is thrown at our energy disposal in blood.

When an organism feels energy drained, body and mind crave addictively for glucose... No matter what type of glucose if depleted it needs some instant fix. All cells feel truly dying if they don't get it. Out of glucose you are out of energy for the works of your liver, brains, breathing, digesting talking thinking, etc. This is the type of feeling of thousands of overweight people. They fill dying and their body demand glucose in food form immediately. They feel so energy drained that can not wait to use a complex food such as a protein or a complex carbohydrate. Also fat people were trained by parents and relatives to sub sane this cravings with desserts, cookies sodas, etc. So you are right when you are hungry no matter how much food you take 30 minutes ago. There is a real biological base for it! This is because your Candida and yeasts had consumed all glucose you take before.

So reviewing this process.: If you have to much yeasts and Candida in your digestive system As you take more sugar or quick glucose food (breads, pancakes, candies sodas, etc.) you feed first these parasites and they grow quickly. At the same time they eat from your food precisely what you are trying to get: Energy, your energy via quick glucose.

The instant fix becomes some bread a cookie or soda or something mostly sugar sweetened. Being sugars one chemical step from glucose how can be explained that someone who ate a lot of sugar can be hypoglycemic and energy drained? The energy contained in 3 cakes with ice cream chocolate and coke is the same as 10 big steaks! Calories contained in that meal will be enough for others to live several days.

Where is all that energy consumed? Where does that energy go? The answer is that simple sugars are consumed first by our Parasites mainly Candida and yeast. That process transforms energy in alcohol, CO_2 and then any rest of glucose is used by our body. To get out of cravings we eat this kind of stuff in excess

Overweight people are starving with their stomach full of food!

Their body craves for glucose because there is none or very little glucose remaining in their blood (hypoglycemia). How is this? Remember that is not the food you eat what nourishes you is the food that you can digest and put into you blood stream! After eating lot of carbs and sugars, yeast and Candida eat all the sugar in our guts, grow and leave us hypoglycemic.

The feeling of glucose absence is equal to feel in state of dying.

A simple way to get glucose it is from refined sugar and breads; the problem is that this kind of food is first consumed by Candida and yeast. As more simple sugars are eaten more millions of colonies are fostered in our guts.

Yeast and Candida are nurtured by simple sugars from cookies bread and all kind of food with added sugars (90% of available products in counters). A big percent of all food in supermarkets are composed of that. All of them increase sugars in your digestive system but you know who eat most of it? : Yeast and Candida. So guess what? You start growing big colonies in your gastrointestinal Tract. As far as more sugar you bring to the table Candida grow exponentially. They start demanding you more and more sugars, because sugar and simple starches are their main nutrient. Candida and yeast eat our remaining glucose not allowing glucose to enter the blood stream. Candida are the first to eat the sugars you put in your table. So what happens then?

We feel starving because we actually are starving.

Due to these parasites people are always the verge of hunger, hypoglycemia and hypo-tension. That means Candida bring blood glucose levels to the bottom and so is our body energy. So there is an immediate need of something quick to cure hunger and cravings. In that stage any person will eat any available food with quick glucose availability. Is a fight for survival.

How the fat comes to play:

In this stage overweight people eat simple sugars in excess to feed themselves and their parasites. That means eating a lot becomes a survival mechanism starts to operate: Trying to override the feeling of hunger we start eating in excess..

What Happens when Eating big portions become the Norm?

Eating in excess makes blood sugar level concentration boom. By a homeostatic regulation   Pancreas star secreting insulin to lower glucose   when   blood concentration reaches over certain threshold. Insulin converts glucose in fat. This way our body converts simple sugars and starches in fat and this fat is send to our fat deposits: belly hips legs, etc.

Please observe that If you eat sugars you make fats if you eat fat you do glicolisis (glucose in blood)

Excess of sugar makes pancreas secrete insulin. All excess of sugar processed via insulin becomes fat. Guess what type of fat? Low density fat which is the culprit of our clogged arteries Most of fat made by this process becomes low density cholesterol (LDL or bad and sticky cholesterol) Eating sugars excessively makes your pancreas overwork when making lots of insulin to lower sugar excess in blood and Diabetes may occur. Later There is an adrenal response that is another stage of glucose-insulin deregulation too much adrenaline is produced to compensate hyperinsulinism —a state of adrenergic hyper-vigilance. And this means stress and exhaustion.

Yeast and Candida

Yeast and Candida overgrow has been neglected and considered a minus problem and they are not.

Candida is a big problem and underlines our actual civilization.

Have you feed wild birds with those supermarket packs? If you have done so you'll remember that in a place where there were not any birds suddenly they show up hundreds of them waiting to be fed. As long as you feed them in a daily basis there will be a lot of them. If you travel in the ocean and start throwing discarded food to the water You'll have hundreds of sharks after you.

There is a natural homeostatic response to abundance: the compensatory grow of predators of such abundance.
For example if there is a dead cat in a park you will notice that there is a bad odour at the beginning. This attracts many small predators that later , if the cat is not removed you will notice that all cat's flesh is totally consumed by zillions of bacteria and parasites which act like environment cleaners. And, when the labour is finished they leave or die of hunger.

The same happens with parasites if you feed them the perfect food they will boom by hundredth fold. Candida and yeast thrive on sugars and simple carbohydrates that mean that each time you eat more sugar or breads you feed them and boost millions of colonies in your digestive system.

These yeast and Candida colonies will demand more sugar and will take most of the sugar off your system making you feel weak and hungry again

Our food culture is based in breads and these are made with yeast and sugars , Candida preferred food are breads and sugars. They are the ones (Candida) who crave for sugars. And they make you crave for them as well. As more you eat sugars and bread whole colonies will grow within you and all of them will need more sugar to be fed. That's why after you ate you need sugar or dessert again...

Go inside a supermarket and observe how many of all shelves are used to help us feed our gut carried Yeast and Candida. It looks that all the supermarket system works for feeding them! Breads cookies, sodas and all kind of pastas and starches help us breed them. All meals with sugar added! All juices with sugar added. Additionally, each time you have flu or any infection you get antibiotics which kill your healthful GI (gastrointestinal) bacteria in charge of controlling yeasts overgrown.

The average adult has more than three pounds of beneficial bacteria in the GI tract. These bacteria help us digest food and provide the B vitamins necessary for life and for metabolic energy. They keep harmful microbes from killing us. When we overfeed our yeasts beneficial bacteria is dominated by these parasites. And things become worst for our friendly bacteria if we add antibiotics.

Parasites live in a world where there are many other enemies including our friendly bacteria like lactobacillus acidophilus

Chlorine

Chlorine in water is another enemy of our natural beneficial bacteria it kill many and yeasts and Candida are practically immune to this level of chlorine. If you take municipal water I recommend you to take it out and leave it open or boil it to get rid of chlorine.

Antibiotics

Any antibiotics that you take will kill plenty of your GI tract friendly bacteria mostly lactobacillus, yeast and Candida will grow tenth fold. Antibiotics are one of the leading causes of Candida overgrowth. There are many studies that demonstrate a quick imbalance between friendly bacteria and Yeasts after taking any Antibiotics.

Stress

Stress reduces your energy to combat yeast. As in any conflict if one of the contenders is weak looses the battle

Yeast and Candida are almost the same type of fungus they have in common same kingdom, Sub-phylum, class, order, and family. They act almost in the same way. You can see here both share the same:

Kingdom:	Fungi
Phylum:	Ascomycota
Subphylum:	Saccharomycotina
Class:	Saccharomycetes
Order:	Saccharomycetales
Family:	Saccharomycetaceae

Candida are not a simple thing they colonize our major energy organs like pancreas and liver and increase our chances or becoming extremely overweight.

Symptoms of a Candida Overgrowth

Signs of overgrowth and the progression of spreading yeast are very similar: Candida has been implicated in prostatitis and prostate cancer in men and vaginal yeast infections in women. Candida symptoms include indigestion, lethargy, food and environmental allergies, joint soreness, jock itch, depression, dry, itchy, flaky skin, anxiety, recurring irritability or mood swings, heartburn, chest pain, acne or other skin problems, migraine headaches, recurring cystitis/vaginal infections, premenstrual tension, menstrual problems and fungal infections of the nails. Candida move through the tract shared by the reproductive and urinary systems. Males have contracted it Candida infection after oral sex with an infected female. For this reason it is common that males end up with the spores in their lungs! Thus bypassing the normal route taken by Candida to invade the body.

Yeast an Candida toxins

Yeasts produce a by-product called acetaldehyde, a toxic substance resulting in several health consequences. In fact, acetaldehyde is the compound that produces the symptoms in an alcohol "hang-over." Molybdenum plays a role as a cofactor in helping break down acetaldehyde to a form that actually provides the body with energy.* Molybdenum plays a large role in the detoxification pathway for acetaldehyde in the human body. There are dozens of known toxins released be yeast in the body. Candida infection overwork the liver the pancreas the adrenal glands and the immune system as the body tries to detoxify these poisons.

Conclusions:

- ### Cause of hunger = Parasites + sugar

Our craving and binges come from thriving parasites from our gastrointestinal tract. We nurture them with sugars and simple carbohydrates

- ### To Get Rid of Parasites= change our GI environment

We must get rid of this parasites and the only real way is doing it by exhaustion. We should take something that can restore the normal bacteria and exhaust parasitic action.

First not eating more yeast, secondly not feeding them and nurture them. this is the first stage that we will do in our Program.

How to cut feeding Sugars and Simple Carbs to our Parasites

There is another main problem here. We know that there are Parasites addict to sugars dominating our life and nutrition. Making a kind of voodoo and making us eat what we know we must not eat. Breaking our will and convincing us of anything that take us to break our rules. How can we can get out of this circle?

Correct Food and Nutrients

I'll show what are the main Nutrients that will feed us and not our Parasites
We will take nutrients that will help us reactivate our metabolism. Liver and kidneys organs are the most inactivated by the toxic debris of these parasites.

Helping Supplements

There are several supplements that act like a miracle over cravings. You will learn how and when to use them.

Supplements:

Thermogenic supplements:

- **green tea**

- **mustard**

- **coffee**

- **Fish Oil**

- **Enzymes**

- **Apple cider**

- **Aloe Vera**

- **VITAMIN C**

- **Calcium:**

- **PH Balance**

- **calcium issue**

- **Choline inositol factor**

- **Zinc Selenium Magnesium Manganese**

- **Iodine**

Forbidden Foods and Drugs

- **Sugars**

- **any kind of breads**

- **Regular Sodas**

- **Chlorine**

- **Antibiotics**

Remember when was the last time you take antibiotics or chlorinated water. Both things are part of the regular American life.

Candida symptoms:

Signs differ from individual to individual and change in intensity, or might come and go. Many signs are unseen, which can make it hard for others to realize the great array of devastating signs and symptoms with which we all deal.
The most frequent are:

- *a great incapacitating exhaustion*

- *problems with awareness and short-term memory space*

- *influenza-like signs such as soreness in the joint parts and muscle tissue*

- *intense rigidity in the shoulder blades and throat*

- *hyper-acidity/acid flow back*

- *brown coloured mucus in the back of the throat*

- *blisters in the mouth/tongue/throat*

- *either white or "blood blisters"*

- *un-refreshing sleep*

- *sore throat*

- *white coated tongue*

- *dark circles under the eyes*

- *an aversion in order to getting touched or bouncing*

- *"crawling" skin*

- *chronic sinus problems and headaches including migraines*

- *chronic dental problems*

- *Visual disruptions may consist of blurring, level of sensitivity to mild and eye discomfort.*

Psychological problems may include:

- *depression*

- *irritability*

- *anxiety*

- *panic attacks*

- *recurring obsessive thoughts*

- *personality changes and mood swings (irrational rage or crying for no reason - fear of talking to people, any kind of confrontation, isolation)*

- *paranoia*

- *chills and night sweats*

- *shortness of breath*

- *dizziness and balance problems*

- *sensitivity to heat and/or cold*

- *alcohol intolerance*

- *gluten and/or casein intolerance*

- *irregular heartbeat*

- *irritable bowel*

- *constipation and/or diarrhoea*

- *painful gas and abdominal bloating*

- *low-grade fever or low body temperature*

- *numbness, tingling and/or burning sensations in the face or extremities*

- *dryness of the mouth and eyes*

- *difficulty swallowing*

- *projectile vomiting*

Also:

- *menstrual problems including PMS and endometriosis*
- *recurrent yeast infections*
- *recurrent ear infections*
- *rashes and dry, flaking skin*
- *eczema*
- *dermatitis*
- *acne*
- *epidermis discoloration and/or blotchiness*
- *dry skin*
- *jock and rectal itching*
- *chronic athlete's foot*
- *chronic toenail and fingernail fungus*
- *ringing in the ears (tinnitus)*
- *allergies and sensitivities to noise/sound, foods, odours, chemicals*
- *anaemia*
- *weight changes without changes in diet*
- *light-headedness*
- *feeling in a fog*

- *fainting*
- *muscle twitching and muscle weakness*
- *restless leg syndrome*
- *low sex drive and/or numbness in the genital area"*

With so many folks struggling, the doctors couldn't clean our signs away forever. Many more people are now being diagnosed with Chronic Fatigue Syndrome , Chronic Fatigue and Immune Dysfunction, Fibromyalgia symptoms , Lupus, Hypothyroidism, Leaky Gut Syndrome, Crohn's Disease, Irritable Bowel Syndrome, Celiac Disease, chronic sinusitis, atopic eczema, Seborrheic Dermatitis, Tinea Versicolor, GI dysbiosis, adrenal dysfunction, Rosacea, Psoriasis, Macular Degeneration, Barrett's Esophagus, Lactose Intolerance, Gluten and/or Casein Intolerance, Meniere's Disease, Obsessive Compulsive Disorder , and sometimes just depression which can accompany many disease states).

It may be an fundamental condition in numerous conditions, but is usually not necessarily diagnosed, misdiagnosed, disputed to even exist or is disregarded altogether. The number of children born with Autism 30 years ago was approximately 1 in 500,000. The rough number today is an incredible 1 in 166. Alzheimer's disease alone has already been forecasted to crack our health care program in the following 20 years.[2]

The risks of Candida Overgrowth. Candida actually, in its yeast form and in being in proportion with proper amounts of beneficial bacteria it is beneficial. We all have this form of Candida in our bodies in some amounts. The Candida population should be low and indiscernible. "Friendly" bacteria and a healthy immune system prevent this yeast from over colonizing the GI tract and becoming an infectious fungus.

An antibiotic will only make the yeast growth worsen. Antibiotics are meant to kill of harmful bacteria, but they also kill off our beneficial bacteria as well. The average adult has three pounds of beneficial bacteria in the GI tract and we have formed a symbiotic relationship with them. These Bacteria help us digest food and provide the B vitamins necessary for life. They also keep harmful microbes from killing us.

Unfortunately, when we take an antibiotic, drink chlorinated water or eat a diet with lots of sugar and acid, the beneficial bacteria are killed off and yeast is quick to take advantage by over colonizing. Some of the Candida can then change from

---

[2]   Cf htp://www.dfwcfids.org/cfids/index.shtml or http://www.naturalhealingpro.com/candida-ease-homeopathy-new.html

the yeast form to the fungal form. According to a research pioneer, C. Orian Truss, MD, in a paper published in a 1978 issue of The Journal of orthomolecular Psychiatry, Candida Albicans proliferates in the intestines because of several factors, including stress, lowered immune system, antibiotic overuse, oral contraceptives, and use of cortisone or prednisone"[3] He forgot to add what we have said here: Sugar main food for Parasites

STRATEGIC STAGED ABUNDANT HUNGER FREE TRIPLE MONODIET

The goal of this Program

The goal of this Program is to control our Candida and bring them back to a normal minimum stage by not overfeeding

---

[3]Check http://www.wholeapproach.com/candida/treatment.php or http://www.nutrition2000.com/Candida/default.asp

them. This way we will get rid of our cravings and abnormal hunger.

After controlling parasites in our body by our Program .We have to find a way to reactivate our liver pancreas, our kidney and thyroid functions lowered by toxins segregated by these same parasites. Of course all made only with the natural resources of food and their properties. The naughty feeling of being weak and fatigued is due to slow metabolism due to toxic liver and thyroid inactivation.

We need energy to get rid of fat water and inflammation also of large amounts of waste retained in our tissues due to toxins, hyperinsulinemia and excessive stress.

Strategic:

Food selected for this Program is picked because the synergistic relation they have with our body. They are high energy radiant food that will allow you to break your inertia.

Staged

Each meal must be separated from the others and each of them has a special goal within the Program. It can be for your liver cleansing or designed for your stomach to do proper digestive exercise or for promoting fat metabolism.

Abundant

Portions are abundant and they will make easy for you to follow. This Program is not going to kill you of famine. It will give enough energy to your body for shedding your fat and water, getting out of inflammation due to parasites and bloating.

Most important of lose weight you'll shed size and get more density. Overweight people have low density.

Hunger free

You may eat a lot at the beginning and you will cut portions as you feel comfortable. No matter this you will succeed if you follow trough.

All of the food we put in this pages is necessary all of them have a reason and must not be neglected. Portions are important but in our case they are big portions because our goal is to kill our cravings and we will start by eating big portions of STRATEGIC food and you must take it no matter you don't feel very comfortable at the beginning.

The Order

This is a staged Program. With this we mean that the order in the way you eat your meals is very important. Breakfast is the most important food in the day. If I ask you to eat a Salad in the morning you must eat it. and within the size parameters you can eat a bigger portion but not a lesser amount.

Size of portions

The goal is to reduce without hunger, so the size of the portion is very important because is fighting against your hunger, and related to your extended stomach. Remember you are eating strategic food. This food will work in favour of your hunger or your liver or your metabolism.

If you can eat any portion you want of any of the allowed foods. YOU MUST NOT EAT NOT PERMITTED FOOD you will have availability of food and snacks that you can get in any store. So you don't have excuse!

Salad Components:

Salad components including the dressing are crucial and strategic, put all or most of the components. If really any of these ingredients you can not eat avoid it. But please! Make your best effort!
All of them are good but combined are marvellous...

Shopping list:

Get all thermogenic agents mentioned in page 88.

Salads:

why Salads?
Salads are important for many reasons. First of all they have chelated water in them.

In all salad as other shopping list ingredients certified organic is recommended but regular will be ok.

Almonds (toasted or raw)

Avocado
Cucumbers
Eggs
Organic Coconut Oil
Extra Virgin Olive Oil
Garlic cloves
Italian peppers
Jalapeño peppers
Peppers (red green and yellow)
Plain Low fat yoghurt
Sea salt (please don't use regular salt)
Spring mix
Tomatoes

Fruits:
The cheaper fruits in stores are usually the better because they are at the season's best. They are abundant and in their best state
Avoid watermelons and cantaloupes
We recommend oranges grapes pineapple and apples

Meats and Proteins

Find the best place around to get the freshest cuts available. I strongly recommend grass fed
livestock.

You can pick between

Chicken
All game bird
Almonds and nuts
Beef
Beef
Beverage
Cornish Hen
Duck
Egg
Goose
Lamb
Lamb
Pheasant
Quail
Rabbit
Salmon
Squirrel
Tofu
Tuna
Turkey
Yoghurt Plain
Veal
Goat Whey

Snacks:

These are snacks you can get in almost any convenience store
Try to get your snack from a fresh source provider
Almonds
Cashew Nuts
Sesame seed
Safflower seed
If you have more than 2 ½ hours of having a meal you can snack:

Grapes
Oranges
Papaya
Apple

These are snacks you can get in almost any convenience store

Supplements:

Fish Oil: 4000 mg a day
Digestive Enzymes: The most necessary come in a one bottle
Pancreatin (protease, amylase, lipase),Ox Bile Extract,
Diastase, Papain Cellulase, Bromelain, Betaine, HCl

Aloe Vera in natural leafs

Take 1 inch of Aloe Vera leaf cut out the green portion and
eat the crystal part if you don't want to chew it you may put
it firs in the blender with a fruit. Is great at inflammation and
has a powerful anti-parasites effect with a totally gentle and
soothing action

After that take calcium (800 mg) and wait at least 30 minutes
before taking any meal.
VITAMIN C

During a diet the body is compromised by many oxidant
processes and toxins, So for detoxification is necessary to
take a good amount of vitamin C. Vitamin C is the main
source of health you can get to with any kind of side effects.
I want to refer you to the vitamin c foundation in relation to
the optimum dose of vitamin c:

"How Much Is Too Much?

The Secret to Lose Weight, Stop Your Cravings

and Flatten Your Belly in a Snap

Dr. Robert Cathcart believes the ideal intake for any individual is the highest level they can tolerate without loose bowels. On the basis of his experience with 11,000 patients over 14 years this bowel tolerance level may be 10 to 15 grams in a healthy person, 30 to 60 grams in a person with a cold, and over 199 grams per day in a person with a serious infectious illness. During an infectious illness the best clinical results have been achieved by maintaining high vitamin C levels in the blood through 3 or more grams every four hours."

Thankfully, Ascorbic acid is probably the least toxic materials that you can buy. 4 studies offered 10 grams regarding ascorbic acid to around 3000 patients with out an individual documented likelihood associated with poisoning. Besides the bowels. Actually, there has not been a unitary circumstance of poisoning resulting from getting vitamin C supplements, regardless of unfounded reviews regarding potential threat for kidney stones, elevating blood vessels uric acid levels, or chronic scurvy. It really is not likely in which virtually any vitamin has been analyzed in order to this extent regarding toxicity and it is secure to assume that Additional levels of at least ten grams each day, or as much as colon threshold, are totally risk-free. "[4]

---

[4]http://www.vitamincfoundation.org/mega_1_1.html

"WHAT IS OPTIMUM

"Whichever way you look at it the figures come out in the same ballpark. The optimum intake is likely to be in the region of 1,000 mg (1 gram) to 10,000 mg (10 grams) per day, if you are in the grips of cardiovascular disease, an infectious or immune system disease, or cancer the ideal level may be much higher. If you drink excessive amounts of alcohol, live in a polluted city, have a stressful lifestyle, take drugs including aspirin, or smoke, your optimal intake will again be raised. An intake of 200 to 300 mg of vitamin C per day is required to raise the average smoker's vitamin C level to that of a non-smoker. An intake of around 50 mg per cigarette probably affords maximum protection. "[5]

Contrary to man, animals can synthesize vitamin C and these are the amounts they produce in a daily basis:

Vitamin C produced per day by different animal species (equivalent for a 175 lbs Man) [6]

Goat	2,280 - 13,300 mg
Rat	2,737 - 13,902 mg
Rabbit	1,547 - 15,820 mg

[5]ibid

[6]ibid

Cow	1,099 - 1,281 mg
Mouse	2,352 - 19,250 mg
Sheep	1,736 mg
Cat	336 - 2,800 mg

1000mg = 1 gram of Vitamin C.

Calcium:

Take 800 mg starting the day.

SUGAR RELATED PROBLEMS

The result of people feeding with sugar their inner parasites and nurturing has all this ill effects. Learn about them in this list compiled by Dr Mercola.

1. "Sugar can suppress your immune system and impair your defenses against infectious disease.
2. Sugar upsets the mineral relationships in your body: causes chromium and copper deficiencies and interferes with absorption of calcium and magnesium.
3. Sugar can cause can cause a rapid rise of adrenaline, hyperactivity, anxiety, difficulty concentrating, and crankiness in children.
4. Sugar can produce a significant rise in total cholesterol, triglycerides and bad cholesterol and a decrease in good cholesterol.
5. Sugar causes a loss of tissue elasticity and function.
6. Sugar feeds cancer cells and has been connected with the development of cancer of the breast, ovaries, prostate, rectum, pancreas, biliary tract, lung, gallbladder and stomach.
7. Sugar can increase fasting levels of glucose and can cause reactive hypoglycemia.
8. Sugar can weaken eyesight.
9. Sugar can cause many problems with the gastrointestinal tract including: an acidic digestive tract, indigestion, mal-absorption in patients with functional bowel disease, increased risk of Crohn's disease, and ulcerative colitis.
10. Sugar can cause premature aging.
11. Sugar can lead to alcoholism.

12. Sugar can cause your saliva to become acidic, tooth decay, and periodontal disease.
13. Sugar contributes to obesity.
14. Sugar can cause autoimmune diseases such as: arthritis, asthma, multiple sclerosis.
15. Sugar greatly assists the uncontrolled growth of Candida Albicans (yeast infections).
16. Sugar can cause gallstones.
17. Sugar can cause appendicitis.
18. Sugar can cause hemorrhoids.
19. Sugar can cause varicose veins.
20. Sugar can elevate glucose and insulin responses in oral contraceptive users.
21. Sugar can contribute to osteoporosis.
22. Sugar can cause a decrease in your insulin sensitivity thereby causing an abnormally high insulin levels and eventually diabetes.
23. Sugar can lower your Vitamin E levels.
24. Sugar can increase your systolic blood pressure.
25. Sugar can cause drowsiness and decreased activity in children.
26. High sugar intake increases advanced glycation end products (Sugar molecules attaching to and thereby damaging proteins in the body).
27. Sugar can interfere with your absorption of protein.
28. Sugar causes food allergies.
29. Sugar can cause toxemia during pregnancy.
30. Sugar can contribute to eczema in children.

31. Sugar can cause atherosclerosis and cardiovascular disease.
32. Sugar can impair the structure of your DNA.
33. Sugar can change the structure of protein and cause a permanent alteration of the way the proteins act in your body.
34. Sugar can make your skin age by changing the structure of collagen.
35. Sugar can cause cataracts and nearsightedness.
36. Sugar can cause emphysema.
37. High sugar intake can impair the physiological homeostasis of many systems in your body.
38. Sugar lowers the ability of enzymes to function.
39. Sugar intake is higher in people with Parkinson's disease.
40. Sugar can increase the size of your liver by making your liver cells divide and it can increase the amount of liver fat.
41. Sugar can increase kidney size and produce pathological changes in the kidney such as the formation of kidney stones.
42. Sugar can damage your pancreas.
43. Sugar can increase your body's fluid retention.
44. Sugar is enemy #1 of your bowel movement.
45. Sugar can compromise the lining of your capillaries.
46. Sugar can make your tendons more brittle.
47. Sugar can cause headaches, including migraines.

48. Sugar can reduce the learning capacity, adversely affect school children's grades and cause learning disorders.
49. Sugar can cause an increase in delta, alpha, and theta brain waves which can alter your mind's ability to think clearly.
50. Sugar can cause depression.
51. Sugar can increase your risk of gout.
52. Sugar can increase your risk of Alzheimer's disease.
53. Sugar can cause hormonal imbalances such as: increasing estrogen in men, exacerbating PMS, and decreasing growth hormone.
54. Sugar can lead to dizziness.
55. Diets high in sugar will increase free radicals and oxidative stress.
56. High sucrose diets of subjects with peripheral vascular disease significantly increases platelet adhesion.
57. High sugar consumption of pregnant adolescents can lead to substantial decrease in gestation duration and is associated with a two fold increased risk for delivering a small-for-gestational-age infant.
58. Sugar is an addictive substance.
59. Sugar can be intoxicating, similar to alcohol.
60. Sugar given to premature babies can affect the amount of carbon dioxide they produce.
61. Decrease in sugar intake can increase emotional stability.

62. Your body changes sugar into 2 to 5 times more fat in the bloodstream than it does starch.
63. The rapid absorption of sugar promotes excessive food intake in obese subjects.
64. Sugar can worsen the symptoms of children with attention deficit hyperactivity disorder (ADHD).
65. Sugar adversely affects urinary electrolyte composition.
66. Sugar can slow down the ability of your adrenal glands to function.
67. Sugar has the potential of inducing abnormal metabolic processes in a normal healthy individual and to promote chronic degenerative diseases.
68. Intravenous feedings) of sugar water can cut off oxygen to your brain.
69. Sugar increases your risk of polio.
70. High sugar intake can cause epileptic seizures.
71. Sugar causes high blood pressure in obese people.
72. In intensive care units: Limiting sugar saves lives.
73. Sugar may induce cell death.
74. In juvenile rehabilitation camps, when children were put on a low sugar diet, there was a 44 percent drop in antisocial behaviour.
75. Sugar dehydrates newborns.
76. Sugar can cause gum disease."[7]

---

[7] If you want to see al the refernces go to:
http://www.mercola.com/2005/may/4/sugar_dangers.htm

In case you have a strong Candidiasis

you have to follow this strict diet.

Anti-Candida diet

Cut out all of the following:

Sugar, all types: brown, white, syrup, molasses, honey, fructose, lactose, maltose, dextrose etc. Check all tins and packets,
yeast products: bread, pizza, buns, breadcrumbs, marmite, Oxo, Bovril, Bisto, gravy mix etc. flavoured foods i.e. crisps and foods containing citric acid.
Refined grains, white flour products, cakes, biscuit, pasta, cornflour, cereals etc. all prepared breakfast cereals except Shredded Wheat and purpose made options like Kashi
cured and smoked products: bacon, meats, kippers etc.
fermented products, vinegar, pickles, chutney, soya sauce, alcohol
tea, coffee, ovaltine, chocolate, etc and all malted products

cows milk, cheese cream except yogurt and cottage cheese
fruit, fresh, juice or dried (some fresh fruit can be added after
three weeks)
mushrooms
peanuts and peanut products

foods that you can eat

Onions and garlic,
Fresh vegetables and their juices (beware of carrot juice it
contains a lot of sugar) Rainbow salads are good,
Rice cakes, oat cakes (unmalted) ,Ryvita, sesame and original
only,
soya milks, butter, cottage cheese and yogurt.
herbs, mild spices,
freshly cracked nuts, seeds
water, fruit and herb teas
cold pressed oils
Brown rice and flours, use for cakes and pastry, etc.
Oats (porridge makes an excellent breakfast – make with
water and serve with nuts, seeds and yogurt)
meats, unprocessed preferably organic or free-range
fish preferably unprocessed, oily fish is best
eggs, lentils, peas and beans

To replace important nutrients

Take a good multi vitamin and mineral, vitamin C and any other nutrients prescribed by your therapist. At this stage chromium should help to control blood sugar.

To re-colonize the gut

Take probiotics - Lactobacillus acidophilus, bifidus
Take fructo oligo saccherides
Eat natural yogurt daily

To treat the genitourinary tract
Douching with either:
fresh aloe vera juice
propolis tincture
garlic water (crush a clove in water - strain)
insert : yoghurt
aloe vera jelly

To repair the Intestine

Avoid foods that you may be hypersensitive to. Cow's milk and milk products and wheat are usually the most likely here. To cut back the stress on the immune system and to allow the maximum absorption of the nutrients you are advised to combine your foods and to rotate them. An easy explanation of food combining is not to eat proteins and carbohydrates on the same dinner because they are digested in different acidic environments. A rotation diet conditions the basic principle that it takes five days for traces of a food to be removed from the body. Eating a food type only every five days means that:

the immune system has a chance to recover by not being subjected to the same allergens everyday.

when food is re-introduced after five days an adverse re-action will indicate that your body is intolerant to that substance.

Eat plenty of fresh vegetables, organic if possible to provide essential nutrients and antioxidants to repair the immune system and fibre to help repair the digestive system.

Even though complete excess fat usage has not yet altered significantly in the last hundred years, there's been a huge shift through saturated fats consumption to polyunsaturated body fat mostly due to the fact we have been advised It is healthier. A hundred years ago, cancer malignancy charges have been very low. A person's system's body fat make-up is about 55% mono-unsaturated, forty two% over loaded, leading to 3% polyunsaturated excess fat. We actually require almost no polyunsaturated fat within our eating habits. Modern diets can contain as much as 30% of calories as polyunsaturated oils. The best evidence indicates that our intake of polyunsaturated-saturated fats should not be greater than 4% of the caloric total.

The theory behind the increased cancer rates is that polyunsaturated fats can displace saturated fats in cell structures. The problem with polyunsaturated fats is that they are unstable. Especially when in skin cell structures, polyunsaturated fats would be easily damaged by contact with oxygen or by ultraviolet light from the sun, forming what are known as free radicals. In turn, free radicals are known to be able to damage the cell's DNA. This genetic cell damage, blamed on the sun but more appropriately due to excessive polyunsaturated fat in the diet, leads to skin cancer.

PH Balance

Bodily Ph is something that mostly nobody takes in account. Anyone that has taken care of a fish tank knows how important PH is for the health of the aquarium. The same thing happens with what you eat, as more blood acidity forming food you take yeast and Candida will grow exponentially they love acidity and they will thrive in it.

Check your PH in urine and in saliva and check it out after you make this diet. You can even make some blood tests so you can see the changes. Candida is the sign of our food culture. More than 85% of what you have available is mixed with sugar. Why? There are Extra economic powerful reasons. Sugar brings you back to eat compulsively and that multiplied by millions produce trillions. That is why Is so hard to get away of cravings and binges. Here you have a way is up to you to take advantage of it.

Remember here is not the simple solution that many people fall in to. Meat is an alkaline

Simple guide to free yourself from Hunger, Cravings and binges.

This is a simple guide so you can use the secrets you are about to receive and start getting slim immediately.

At the end you'll have mastered the real truth and power to domain your appetite.

Which and where are the food that loot your energy.

How to go against each of your enemies.

Do first

A-Learn which are the Worst enemies of your Body Furnace.

B-Which are your friends food wise

C-How to start, so you can defeat your cravings and constant hunger.

D- Which are your bodyguards

E- How to start this program.

A-Worst enemies of your Body Furnace.

1.- SUGAR AND ANY FOOD THAT CONTAIN IT.

Sugar is easily transformed in glucose. Glucose is the main energy for all cells of all living organisms.

Sugar = Glucose = Main food to living cells.

Sugar is to living organisms as oil is to our Economy

Why then Sugar is your worst enemy?:

Is not because makes LDL (The worst Lipids)

Not because makes you diabetic

Not because it produces or is linked to more than to 70 of the worst illnesses in earth.

The original and starting point is Because: ---- **Sugar is the main food for the main monsters you have inside: CANDIDA and YEAST.**

If you have a Bunch of Hyenas is your backyard and you feed them enormous amounts of meat, they will reproduce and be so many that if you some day don't continue feeding them they will eat you alive!

90% of food in markets is made with sugar. Sugar is food industry's magic ingredient to multiply thedemand and for profits!

Where you find sugar (Food for your Candida)? Enemy No 1?

You find it in 90% of all foods in markets. Almost everything contain it in high numbers.

- Cakes
- Desserts
- Bread
- Sodas
- cookies
- salad dressings.
- Ketchup
- Pasta sauce
- (50 more pages)

- **Read the Labels!**

2- CANDIDA AND YEAST.

These parasites are the main suckers of your energy and their debris and endotoxins provoke hundred of very ugly diseases. They are waiting inside of you expecting to be nurtured. They are animals**. If you feed them (with sugar) they'll grow exponentially and end with your body's Glucose and start your cravings**. They eat and thrive exclusively in sugar. If you put them together they may be the size of a big boa constrictor inside you.

While baking have you seen the Bread expand? That is because Dough is made with two ingredients added, one is yeast the other one is sugar. You add sugar + yeast in bread and see it grow and expand the same as your belly. You eat yeast and sugar cooked bread. You are increasing the amount of parasites in your gut. You add new enemy combatants to the enemies within. Their goal is grab all your energy source: **glucose.**

Glucose is the energy unit of living beings, is like the oil in our economy. You are feeding the ones who take all your energy.

Glucose is the main food for all your organs and cells. You'll feel hungry always when you don't have enough glucose. They eat the same thing you need: your glucose . If you put a lot of sugar (=glucose) they'll grow and keep you hungry.

You need glucose if you don't have it you will be HUNGRY.

Out or low on glucose = you are hungry.

Parasites are eating what you need

Q- How can you take glucose to live without extra feeding them?

A- Eating foods that this Parasites don't know how to extract glucose from it or they don't like to be involved with.

Yeast and Candida thrive in an environment where simple sugars are around, its their main food.

How you become fat?

Overweight people find by experience that when taking larger amounts of sugar (in different foods), their parasites won't be able to eat all of it so they'll be a chunk remaining so their body can get some Glucose and survive.

Over-eating and permanent cravings are your normal response for the loose of glucose in your blood which is taken by parasites.

Increasing Ingested Sugars are split in three:
- 1st part goes to satisfy the parasites.
- 2nd part goes to whatever your body can take from the large shot of sugars you bring to them. (a large coke for example)
- 3rd remaining excess part is converted in fat by liver and Insulin (mostly Bad LDL and VLDL) and saved in our body fat deposits including your arteries.

Next to it, well nurtured parasites reproduce , eat any available glucose and demand you more sugary stuff in larger amount = you get fatter.

That is why you are really hungry,

is not your mind. it's not a flaw in o your brain or mind. Is you, trying to survive with this form of eating.

The problem is that more sugars make them grow in number. Their troop is bigger each time and they eat quicker and finish with your inside glucose. They'll demand larger sugar amounts so you'll need to feed them with more sweet food each time.

More Sugar = More parasites = Less energy in you = more Hunger= more insulin = fatter and tending to diabetes= cpme back to more sugar.

Because you feel hungry and weak, you won't be able to stop eating sugars cakes pastas cookies sodas, desserts and else.

Before this You must put Candida under control.

So sugar is your anti energy food, your power sucker, is the food of your inner parasites: Candida and yeast.

Sugar >>> Nurture Candida >>> Candida eat glucose >>> you are hungry >> you eat excess sugars >>> insulin makes bad fat (LDL)>>> the cycle starts again while you get fat.

3- BREADS (Cakes and cookies)

WHAT bread has bad for your energy.

3.1- Has bromide

WHAT BROMIDE DOES TO YOU

bromide >>is a poison>> goes inside your thyroid and pituitary >>> your energy slows and you become tired.

Almost all big mills added to flour as a dough conditioner.

3.2-Has yeast

WHAT YEAST DOES TO YOUR BODY? (Already discussed above.)

It brings millions of more highly reproductive glucose eaters they are tight relatives to Candida and live from sugar also. They are almost the same parasite. Also Candida metabolism produce many toxins and excretions that are highly toxic and can bring Cancer and many systemic illnesses.

3.3-Sugar already discussed

If only you can cut sugar and breads from your diet you would be thin as a hair.

But:

Parasites take it all available and and put you out of sugars. This makes you hungry and make you desire to eat. How can you fix this problem? Will see it in the solutions.

4- WATER

Water is bad if contains

4.1- Fluoride poison and thyroid inhibitor. They even add it to bottled water and sodas.

4.2-Chloride poison and thyroid inhibitor. They even add it to **bottled water** and **sodas**

The only water that doesn't contain these toxics is distilled water. You may add sea salt to it to keep up with good minerals.

5- GRAINS

THEY CONTAIN BROMIDE TROUGH PESTICIDES AND as they are BLEACHED

bromide >>is a poison>> goes inside your thyroid and pituitary >>> your energy slows and you become tired and get fat.

CHLORIDE When bleached with potassium bromate or chlorine dioxide
THEY ARE NATURAL WATER ACCUMULATORS in tissue.

RANCHERS KNOW THAT IF THEY WANT THEIR LIVESTOCK TO GAIN WEIGHT THEY HAVE TO INCREASE GRAINS.

Some grains you may eat are gluten free, they are not parasite prone. like

Amaranth, buckwheat, millet, quinoa, Sorghum.

Those grains should be eaten Organic if possible.

6- VEGETABLES and fruits with Pesticides

ALMOST ALL REGULAR VEGETABLES CONTAIN Potassium bromide BROMIDE

bromide >>is a poison>> goes inside your thyroid and pituitary >>> your energy slows and you become tired and get fat.

Vegetables are treated with Potassium bromide should be eaten Organic if possible.

Not all people can find or buy organic; Here are an easy and efficient way to lower your pesticide substance exposure.
Wash your own fruits as if you rinse your hands: petrochemical businesses make pesticides with a chemical sticker which can be insoluble in water. Detergent is more effective getting rid of pesticide residues You can demonstrate this particular on your own. Take large couple of vegetables and place them with dish-water and washing detergent. Combine the cleaning agent inside completely. Carefully watch the water. You will observe proof that detergent operates. Rinse carefully. Now you convert an enemy of your energy in a friend.

Here is a list of the most dangerous and need to wash if not organic:

1-Apples

2-Celery

3-Strawberries

4-Peaches

5-Spinach

6-Nectarines

7-Grapes – imported

8-Sweet bell peppers

9-Potatoes

10-Blueberries – domestic

11-Lettuce

12-Kale/collard greens

The less dangerous are:

1. Onions
2. Sweet Corn
3. Pineapples
4. Avocado
5. Asparagus
6. Sweet peas

7. Mangoes
8. Eggplant
9. Cantaloupe - domestic
10. Kiwi
11. Cabbage
12. Watermelon
13. Sweet potatoes
14. Grapefruit

7- HORMONES

FEMALE HORMONE (Estrogen) ARE GIVEN TO CATTLE OR POULTRY FOR INCREASING THEIR NET WEIGHT AND IS JUST WHAT THEY DO IN YOU. Most Non organic milk meat and poultry have estrogens including some plants. Estrogenic food tends to make you fat and slow. The solution: buy organic.

8- ANTIBIOTICS

When you take antibiotics you kill the friendly bacteria that helps control biologically your Candida and yeast which will flourish with them. If you had taken some less than 3 years previous you need to take probiotics. Look for a probiotic with more than 5 billion organisms per capsule.

9- ARTIFICIAL SWEETENERS.

They have a lot of bad research results, including cancer tumours and organ disease . The worst is that if you wish to be free for life you have to be free of sugar and sweet cravings. These prolong your desire and your memory of this disease.

B- YOUR FRIENDS FOOD WISE

Friends no 1

1- Helpful teas to control cravings due to Parasites.

1.1 Cassia senna tea It will change your gut ecology and will flush your lymphatic system and many parasite toxic debris. It will help you to be out of hunger. "Do not use this product if you have abdominal pain or diarrhea. Consult a healthcare provider prior to use if you are pregnant or nursing. Senna tea is an Asian shrub that grows in India, Pakistan, and China as a mild laxative. Senna tea has a diuretic and laxative effect that acts of natural form eliminating the excesses of fats and toxins, not letting you intake them. Put a bag in a cup, leave it in rest for 5 minutes.

1.2 Bark tea/Cascara sagrada tea. stimulates increased wavelike contractions of the large intestine. Cascara has also been known to expel parasites through its wavelike actions in the lower intestines and is highly recommended for parasite removal. It is anti-viral. Cascara Sagrada is considered one of the safest laxatives and is useful in detoxifying the colon. "Do not use this product if you have abdominal pain or diarrhoea Consult a healthcare provider prior to use if you are pregnant or nursing.

1.3 Green tea. has been a medicine within China and Taiwan not less than 4,000 years. Nowadays, medical investigation both in Asia and the western offers hard proof for the advantages long associated to drinking green tea. It has all kind of antioxidant properties and as well against The trypanocidal action of *green tea* catechins against two different parasites. These purified compounds lysed more than 50% of the *parasites* present in the blood.

1.4 Boldo tea The Boldo tree is local to Chile.
The most typical use of Boldo Leaf teas is actually to cleanse the liver. Boldo leaf provides attributes that assist cleanse the bloodstream when the kidneys or liver are not functioning well. It also helps remove the bile that has gathered in the gall bladder.

1.5 Mate Tea Mate tea includes several minerals and vitamins important to human wellness, which includes nutritional vitamins The Beta-carotene, B1, B2, C and At the, as well as phosphorus, straightener and calcium.

2. Antioxidants and anti carcinogens
3. Yerba Mate green tea

consists of considerable levels of polyphenol anti-oxidants, and it has a rather increased de-oxidising capability as compared to teas. On average, Mate tea consists of ninety two mg of de-oxidising chlorogenic acid for each gram of dried out leaves, no catechins, giving it a significantly higher antioxidant profile than other teas. In-vivo and in-vitro studies are showing that Yerba Mate exhibits significant cancer-fighting activity. In 1995, research at the University of Illinois found Yerba Mate to inhibit the proliferation of oral cancer cells. Chlorogenic acid is marketed under the tradename Svetol as a food active ingredient used in coffee, chewing gum, and mints to promote weight reduction. Chlorogenic acid reduces hepatic transformation of glycogen into glucose and the absorption of new glucose. In addition, in vivo studies on animal subjects have demonstrated that chlorogenic acid lessens the hyperglycaemic peak.[8]

4. Coffee w/o sugar

Friends no 2

---

[8]Clifford, M. N.; Johnston, K. L.; Knigh, S.; Kuhnert, N. (2003). "Hierarchical Scheme for LC-MSn Identification of Chlorogenic Acids

2- Natural High Thermogenic Foods

Thermogenesis is the process of heat production in organisms. Fat needs more heat to be melted and used as energy.

There are two types of cell respiration and metabolic heat generation. One is anaerobic that is made by fermentation. When you have a big and inflated belly and eat mostly carbs, refined grains, bread, sodas and a lot of sugars your guts are a fermenting sac and are promoting anaerobic cell respiration which produces alcohol inhibits your insulin , is prone to cancer and energy wise is 15 times less energetic that Aerobic respiration. This low heat energy production can't melt and metabolise fat.

Food w/Higher thermogenic effect = quicker weight-loss

Bread, grains, sugar, Candida have an anti-thermogenic action against your metabolism.

You need more heat to burn fat than to burn carbs. You'll increase your inner furnace with a choose of thermogenic food-supplements to increase the basal metabolic rate, and thereby increasing the energy expenditure.

- **Hot Peppers**

Capsaicin, a compound found in cayenne, Habanero peppers and most chile peppers raise your body temperature.

- **Mustard:** has special fat burning and body metabolic stimulating properties. You must use it in your path to become hunger free. You should use is sparingly all over your proteins. Candida parasites are animals and they can't stand it.
  It will mask your food's energy so you can use it, not them. You'll be amazed of how your craving disappear using it.[9] Use Dijon Mustard mixed with the regular one. using it.
- **Cassia Senna tea** has an anti yeast and anti Candida action

---

[9] it was shown that certain minor constituents of the diet such as caffeine and associated methylxanthines in tea and coffee could have a profound effect on metabolic rate. The consumption of alcohol was also shown to increase metabolic rate (Rosenberg & Durnin, 1978). The work described in this paper reports the effect of another minor constituent of food, spices, on metabolic rate. Although the use of spices in our food has steadily increased with time little information exists on their effect on the metabolic rate. It has been estimated that approximately 40 different spices are used in our diet today. This communication reports the effect of chilli (red pepper, capsicum annuum) and mustard (Brassica juncea).

- **Green tea** is a non side effect thermogenic and antioxidant tea, plus will have you all day without hunger

- Mate tea-It will give you concentration, power and loss of cravings

- **Coffee w/o sugar** has high thermogenic and antioxidant properties also acts as a appetite suppressant.

- Apple cider Vinegar it will dissolve your fat like magic. Use it in your salads.

- **Garlic has cleaning and antiparasitic action.**

  If you can't stand their smell is due to excess parasites. !Is not you is them: they don't like it!

- **Green Coffee Bean extract.** It'll give you energy stamina and keep you out of hunger

- **Aloe Vera leaf** : Take 1 inch of Aloe Vera in the mornings leaf cut out the green portion and eat the crystal part if you don't want to chew it you may put it first in a blender. Has high anti-parasite and anti-inflammatory action.

- **Gurmar (Gymnema Sylvestre)**
  Gurmar, is often referred to as "sugar destroyer" and has been used in Ayurveda since the 6th century BC. It has been used in Ayurvedic medicine for several centuries as a safe and natural approach to help

regulate sugar metabolism. The key component of Gymnema - Gymnemic Acids - mimics glucose molecules, numbing receptor sites on the tongue. Gymnema contains Gymnemic acid, Quercitol, Lupeol, Beta-Amyrin and Stigmasterol, all of which are thought to help the body maintain healthy blood glucose levels.

- **Lean proteins**

  All lean proteins have a thermogenic effect in metabolism

  - Chicken
  - All game bird
  - Almonds and nuts
  - Beef
  - Beef
  - Beverage
  - Cornish Hen
  - Duck
  - Egg
  - Goose
  - Lamb
  - Lamb
  - Pheasant
  - Quail

- Rabbit
- Salmon
- Squirrel
- Tofu
- Tuna
- Turkey
- Yoghurt Plain
- Veal
- Goat Whey
ACTIVE

Friends no 3

3- Thermogenic Salad Dressings:

The secret of thermogenic dressing is the secret of losing weight with enjoyment. Here is a thermogenic dressing keep it in your fridge and can added to anything you wish.

2 cups of Apple cider vinegar
4 stripped and crushed garlic cloves
2 or 3 soup spoons of mustard

1600 mg of green coffee bean extract.
Crushed jalapeños or 2 Chipotle peppers w/juice.
Sea Salt and olive oil to taste.

Friends no 4

4-Vegetables and Salads.

You could never go wrong taking salads. They'll nurture you they are not easy glucose for parasites. The secret of Salads are dressings You can surround them with many anti-Candida and thermogenic add ons. Always add to your salad a thermogenic dressing like described above.

Why eat salad? Because will fill you with vitamins and minerals, flavonoids antioxidants and it will expand your stomach and make you feel full. Contrary to bloating your stomach by gas expansion; your stomach will have the opportunity to work and muscle out this food in a kind of inner abs work. This salad is not food for Candida or yeast. This meal won't expand nor produce inflammation in your body.

Friend no 5

5-Pure water

Get Distilled water. (don't contains Fluoride or chlorine (both your enemies and powerful poisons.) Only distilled water is out of fluoride, chlorine and Trihalomethanes between all available in the food market. Tap water, sodas and bottled water You can save from very bad diseases only using it. You can add a pinch of sea salt to add good minerals to it. Using your kidney this water will clean many poison you have around stopping you.

Friend no 6.

6-Exercise

Exercise increase your body's thermogenesis as well as cold water. As more aerobic and intense the effect is bigger. They are hundreds of options you can even find plans in you-tube.

Friend no 7.

7-Testosterone boosting foods

Testosterone boosting foods and herbs have a loss weight action.

They are foods such as garlic, onion, celery, radish, almonds, pine nuts, bee pollen, mucuna, ashwaganda and ginseng respectively have shown great impact on sustaining and boosting testosterone, virility, strength and vitality. Also a testosterone booster plant is Fadogia agrestis (Rubiaceae.)

Friend no 8.

8- Hormonal Balancing foods

There are Certain foods and herbs that have shown the capacity to help balance estrogens in the body by inhibiting its formation or by modulating its metabolism. Cruciferous vegetables have this capacity. These foods include **broccoli, cabbage, omega 3 oil, flax, hemp or fish oils, nuts, seeds, turmeric, garlic, onion, oranges, berries, and all greens.**

C- <u>How to start, defeat your Cravings, boost your Energy and Lose Weight?.</u>

After you read about your energy's enemies and friends, you should know you must not take sugars. This means anything that has sweet will go straight to feed and grow your parasites and will keep doing food fermentation instead of oxygen metabolism which is 15 times less energetic. The goal of this information is not tell you only "don't take sugar", but give you the tools and supplements help to quit sugar without hunger and pain"

The first thing you have to do is to clean your gut medium that has become a fermentation tank. Full of parasites waiting so the food gets putrefactive and ferments so you can extract energy from that medium. Getting rid also of the endotoxin secreted by Candida and yeast to gain control of your own body. When you finish this Cassia senna tea, you should use the following teas as a daily help have parasites under control and change your eating habits use them mixed or alternate them they are a great help to keep your parasites at bay.

Bark tea/Cascara sagrada tea

Green tea.

Boldo tea

D-Start here: Flush your parasites

You need to take something that yeast and Candida don't like but that is harmless to your body. Most of candida aggressive medications like Clotrimazole, Miconazole, Tioconazole or Ketoconazole harm your body and prepare it for worst damage. Cassia senna and the other teas mentioned act gently and changes your gut environment. Candida and yeast don't like the substances in those teas.

A-Teas

You need to clean your body of excessive Candida and yeast and for so, you need to flush them. Candida is resistant to antibiotics and lives in relationship to the intestinal environment. When the environment in the intestines changes in ways that do not promote the Candida life and reproductive cycle, they will not continue to live in the same numbers. After flushing them they'll be in much fewer numbers and the remaining will take their normal role in our guts. This is only if you don't start feeding them in the way you had before or take antibiotics.

You should start this program when you feel strong and willing to make a change in your life. Maybe in a weekend when you can use 2 days for your flush and cleaning. If you are not in that stage, wait for this moment to happen.

1ˢᵗ and 2ⁿᵈ days.

Start the day with a Cassia senna tea and you can take from 1-5 cups. If you want to go slowly you can start with ½ cup and increase the amount slowly to at least 3 a day. During the day. This will have very special effects. It will change your gut ecology and will flush your lymphatic system and many parasite toxic debris. It will bring some cramping and loose stools . You can take 1 or 2 cups of Boldo tea that helps clean your liver and gallbladder. Eat lightly during these days . Take a lot of water with a pinch of salt to recuperate liquids. You can add one more day if you feel you haven't drain enough. it's normal that you'll feel a bit weak. After that you'll feel very good.

Senna furthermore should not be consumed by individuals who endure irritable bowel syndrome, Crohns syndrome, ulcerative colitis, anaemia, severe haemorrhoids, blood vessel damage, kidney or liver damage, recent or past colon surgery and by individuals who suffer from colon cancer. In these kinds of cases it is recommended to reduce the use of senna and it will be always wise to check with a doctor concerning the treatment.

If you don't end having a good flush and you feel inflamed, you may try a coffee enema. Agood place to find about it is here

http://www.health-information-fitness.com/coffeeseries.htm

The night of the second day drink one glass of water with a spoon of psillium husk (metamucil or other), that will stabilise your stomach.

3rd day

You will feel very good. You won't feel hungry as always.

take a lot of green tea Green tea during this day.

Teas drinking support

Drink one of the teas or combine them Cassia senna tea, Bark tea/Cascara sagrada tea, Green tea, Boldo Tea, Mate Tea. Take this teas often and as a natural way to control **your parasites, which will try to regain control over yourself**.

How? Craving sweets. Use teas or coffee (no sugar) and you'll be safe.

What to eat: don't take food with sugar added or breads if not you'll start the vicious cycle again. You should eat between vegetables and protein. Later on you may take some fruits but now you have to focus in vegetables and protein using any of your friendly foods.

What to eat at the beginning

- **Proteins** with plenty of mustard. You'll find that eating proteins with mustard will make you feel meal satisfied and out of strong appetite. The reason is that you are hiding the food from your parasites and increasing food's power to produce energy and heat.

- **sweet breaks** If you need a sweet break eat mostly apples or grapefruit. Use your will power. Don 't break to often if possible don't do it before 2 weeks or start. Don't mix food if you take a snack take it as separate in time of a regular meal as possible.

- Salads

  Why eat salad? Because will fill you with vitamins and minerals, flavonoids antioxidants and it will expand your stomach and make you feel full. Contrary to bloating your stomach by gas expansion; your stomach will have the opportunity to work and muscle out this food in a kind of inner abs work. This salad is not food for Candida or yeast. This meal won't expand nor produce inflammation in your body.

- Don't forget to add thermogenic dressing like the one shown above.

Choose a bowl the size of your hunger and change the quantities at taste.

10-20 Almonds (toasted or raw)
½ Avocados
1/3 Cucumber
2 hard boiled eggs
½ sliced Italian peppers
If you like spicy ¼ to 1 Jalapeño raw sliced pepper
1/3 pepper (red green or yellow)
Sea salt (please don't use regular salt)
One to 1 1/2 cups of spring mix or sliced lettuce
1 sliced Tomato
1 spoon of pure coconut oil
1 spoon of Extra Virgin olive oil
2 pressed Garlic cloves
2½ spoons of plain low fat yoghurt or Kefir

Make this question always yourself before you start eating?

Do I feel low energy now and not really hungry? If that is the case

take some tea. If cravings are strong take a fresh apple and eat it slowly, or a protein snack (a piece of beef, chicken. Egg , Tuna etc.)
You are ready and hungry?

Eat.

After a meal is very important you to wait at least 2 hours before taking anything else. That will give your body time to adjust. Take tea or coffee remember no sugar in it or sweeteners. If you crave for something sweet You can eat of the following fruits: grapefruit apples or Papaya (or Papaw, or Carica) You can only eat one of them. Don't mix. The reason is that simple food is easy for your stomach to digest and allows the magic nature has intended in each of its owns recipes. As you eat more combinations is harder for your body to digest and ends doing fat in your body. Fruits are liver friendly. Clean your fruit and eat it all. All fruits must be eaten as whole as possible and the fibre. This will make bulk in your digestive system and will increase your metabolic rate and boost the strength of your liver

Here are some foods you can mix at your taste.

YES FOODS

All friendly foods described here.

All meats(except pork)
Vegetables
Fresh Fruits (mainly apples and grapefruit, After more than a year you can incorporate grapes and oranges)
Eggs
Brown rice, rice cakes (plain) Hot brown rice cereal (plain)

matzos Cookies: they are cookies, they have wheat, but you can take them like a snack and in small amounts. The reason is that they are made with no bleached flour pesticides free, no yeast. Only water. wheat and salt. A water fountain in the desert! You can add small amounts to your salads.

Teas, Coffee.
For cooking or salad dressing: I recommend using cold-pressed olive, coconut, apricot or almond oils (most other oils are toxic to the body).
Seasoning include: Thermogenic dressing (described before) Bragg's Liquid Amino Acids, salt, pepper, etc. (as long as

there are no sugars, yeast, or anything not allowed on this plan.) Naturally raised and organic foods are recommended.

Summary:

These what I have told you is the principles you should use. I won'tt tell you dishes and recipes because I'm sure you know a lot about them. If you are **free of cravings and hunger** don't fall in sugar again. Eat and combine in the amounts you desire as long you are choosing friends not enemies. it's hard to do it but good things in life aren't easy. Take teas all day long if necessary you can make a pot and take it during the day you find that cassia wont produce the strong effects as in your start because parasites are strongly diminished (they will never go completely because they are part of our regular gut environment.

If you are in a restaurant or a Burger King or a Mc Donald's. You can ask for a burger and a salad and take it without the buns. You can add a lot of mustard and protect your meal from parasites. You won't need a lot.

Is hard sometimes. You'll feel like a warrior that defeated a big monster and that's the only truth!